O A P N

OXFORD AMERICAN POCKET NOTES

Coronary Stenting

O A PN

OXFORD AMERICAN POCKET NOTES

Coronary Stenting

By

William D. Brearley, Jr., M.D.
Cardiology Fellow
Division of Cardiovascular Medicine
University of Florida

R. David Anderson, M.D., F.A.C.C.
Associate Professor of Medicine
Director, Interventional Cardiology
Division of Cardiovascular Medicine
University of Florida

Anthony A. Bavry, M.D., M.P.H., F.A.C.C.
Assistant Professor of Medicine
Division of Cardiovascular Medicine
University of Florida

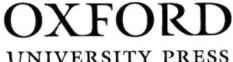

OXFORD
UNIVERSITY PRESS

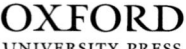
OXFORD
UNIVERSITY PRESS

Oxford University Press, Inc., publishes works that further
Oxford University's objective of excellence
in research, scholarship, and education.

Oxford New York

Auckland Cape Town Dar es Salaam Hong Kong Karachi
Kuala Lumpur Madrid Melbourne Mexico City Nairobi
New Delhi Shanghai Taipei Toronto

With offices in
Argentina Austria Brazil Chile Czech Republic France Greece
Guatemala Hungary Italy Japan Poland Portugal Singapore
South Korea Switzerland Thailand Turkey Ukraine Vietnam

Copyright © 2010 by Oxford University Press, Inc.

Published by Oxford University Press, Inc.
198 Madison Avenue, New York, New York 10016
www.oup.com

ISBN: 978-0-19-973246-3

9 8 7 6 5 4 3 2 1
Printed in the United States of America
on acid-free paper

TABLE OF CONTENTS

INTRODUCTION

The advent and evolution of coronary stenting within the past 25 years is the cornerstone of modern interventional cardiology. Interventional cardiology was born with the first balloon angioplasty by Gruntzig in 1977.[1] This procedure had reasonable outcomes; however, there was a high rate of acute vessel closure and restenosis after balloon angioplasty.[2] This led to the initial development of coronary stents to combat acute vessel closure.[3] Coronary stenting also proved beneficial in treating complications such as dissection and thrombosis after angioplasty, with stents providing a "bail-out" scaffolding with which coronary flow could be restored.[4] Coronary stenting also proved to be efficacious in preventing vessel restenosis compared to balloon angioplasty alone.[5]

The first human stent implantations in peripheral arteries were described by Palmaz et al in 1985.[6] Shortly thereafter, Puel and Sigwart successfully implanted the first stent specifically in a human coronary artery.[3] Complications with these initial efforts mainly involved bleeding associated with anticoagulation. While stents proved very effective periprocedurally, high rates of restenosis remained with this technology. This led to experimentation with various coatings for stents, initially heparin[7] and eventually various antiproliferative agents (referred to as drug-eluting stents). Hence today there are multiple choices available to interventionalists, with the most basic delineation being bare metal stents and drug-eluting stents. Within each broad category there exist multiple stent delivery systems, sizes, structural differences, various metal compositions, and antiproliferative agents for the drug-eluting variety.

There are several controversies currently surrounding coronary stents. Although drug-eluting stents have been proven to decrease vessel restenosis rates compared to bare metal stents,[8] the first-generation drug-eluting stents increased the occurrence of late stent thrombosis, which was uncommon with bare metal stents.[9] Also, stents are being used for multiple types of lesions, many of them considered off-label indications; this calls into question the safety of deploying stents in lesions not exhaustively studied in the initial pivotal trials.[10] Lastly, the duration of dual antiplatelet therapy with aspirin and clopidogrel after stent implantation, especially drug-eluting stents, may need to be extended.[11] Despite these current topics of debate, there is much promise on the horizon of coronary intervention, with bioabsorbable stents and antiproliferative balloons in development.

An understanding of the various principles of coronary stenting, including patient appropriateness, potential complications, and perioperative management, is beneficial to healthcare providers caring for cardiac patients today. Perhaps most importantly, a firm understanding of the importance of dual antiplatelet therapy can have a significant impact on the prevention of stent complications, especially stent thrombosis, which is associated with significant mortality.[12] This guide is meant to serve as a framework for healthcare providers in evaluating patients who may benefit from coronary stenting, as well as properly managing those who are already stent recipients.

STENT CLASSIFICATION

Stent Components and Characteristics

- Since the first human coronary stents were implanted in the mid-1980s, there has been tremendous evolution with regard to fundamental stent composition and design.

- Modern stents are composed of complex metal alloys or high-grade stainless steel, allowing flexibility while still retaining the strength required to maintain vessel patency.
- Stents are available in numerous sizes designated in diameter-versus-length notation—for example, 3.0 mm × 16 mm. This allows deployment in different-length lesions of varying caliber. A typical modern stent is seen in Figure 1.
- Stents from different manufacturers vary with regard to characteristics such as metal composition, strut thickness, hinge point, and cell design, which influences flexibility and maneuverability. Characteristics of an effective coronary stent are noted in Table 1.[13]
- Coronary stents used today can be divided into two major classes: bare metal stents (BMS) and drug-eluting stents (DES).

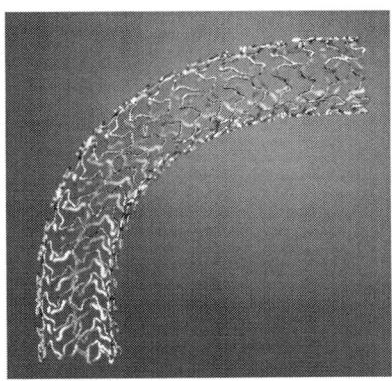

Figure 1 Boston Scientific Liberté bare metal stent

Table 1 Ideal Stent Characteristics

Structural

Flexible/low profile
Radiopaque
Biocompatible
High radial strength
Comfortable
Thromboresistant
Low metal density
Side-branch access
Excellent scaffolding properties

Clinical

Ease of delivery and placement
Low rate of thrombosis
Low rate of restenosis

Adapted from Lau KW, Mak KH, Hung JS, et al. Clinical impact of stent construction and design in percutaneous coronary intervention. *Am Heart J* 2004;147:764–73. With permission from Elsevier.

Bare Metal Stents

- The first coronary stents were BMS and were used to prevent the acute vessel closure that can occur after balloon angioplasty.[5,14] Restenosis is a more subacute problem that develops when a vessel gradually narrows from scar tissue after treatment with a balloon and/or stent. The latter is referred to as in-stent restenosis (ISR).
- Despite the initial success of BMS, they still demonstrated significant ISR, which necessitated repeat procedures.
- While restenosis is a disadvantage of BMS, advantages compared with angioplasty alone include a reduction in acute and subacute vessel closure. They also require a shorter duration of dual antiplatelet therapy with aspirin and clopidogrel (Plavix) (can be as short as 1 month[15]),

mainly due to a low incidence of late thrombotic complications.[9] Because of this, BMS are still frequently used in various circumstances.

- Several BMS are available from multiple manufacturers (Table 2).

Drug-Eluting Stents: First Generation

- The development of DES was an attempt to inhibit the ISR observed with BMS.
- DES are composed of a metal platform, like BMS, but are coated with a polymer impregnated with an antiproliferative agent. These compounds were originally used as chemotherapeutic agents and for immunosuppression after solid organ transplant. The antiproliferative agent is locally released into the vessel wall over time without systemic effects.
- The Cypher (Cordis) and Taxus (Boston Scientific) stents were the first generation of DES; they release sirolimus and paclitaxel, respectively. Food and Drug Administration approval for these devices was obtained after numerous clinical trials showed a significant decrease in ISR compared with BMS.[16,17]
- DES were widely used in the initial years after their approval. Along with increased use came the observation that DES were associated with an increased risk of

Table 2 Bare Metal Stents		
Name	**Manufacturer**	**Composition**
Liberté	Boston Scientific	Stainless steel
Driver	Medtronic	Cobalt–chromium
Multi-link Vision	Abbott	Cobalt–chromium

late (>30 days after implantation) and very late (>1 year) stent thrombosis compared with BMS.[9,18] The incidence was very low, but stent thrombosis was associated with significant morbidity and mortality.[12,19]

- Subsequent large meta-analyses of clinical trials noted the following:
  - An early study found that the rate of very late stent thrombosis was low with DES (5 events per 1,000 patients) but increased when compared with BMS.[9] Extended follow-up revealed no difference in mortality.[20]
  - Stone et al[21] documented that stent thrombosis was more common with both sirolimus and paclitaxel DES compared with BMS; however, there were no significant differences in the rate of death or myocardial infarction with up to 4 years of follow-up.
  - Kastrati et al[22] performed an extensive review of 14 trials comparing sirolimus-eluting stents with BMS. There were no significant differences in the overall risk of death, myocardial infarction, or stent thrombosis with the sirolimus DES compared with BMS; however, there was a small increase in the risk of stent thrombosis with sirolimus stents after the first year of implantation.
- The increased incidence of late and very late stent thrombosis with DES has resulted in the recommendation to lengthen the duration of dual antiplatelet therapy to 12 months.[23]

Drug-Eluting Stents: Second Generation
- Newer antiproliferative agents have gained approval, leading to a second generation of DES (Table 3).
- The second generation of stents are characterized by thinner stent struts, which make them easier to maneuver and potentially cause less endothelial injury upon deployment.

Table 3 Drug-Eluting Stents

Name	Manufacturer	Composition	Antiproliferative Agent	Generation
Cypher	Cordis*	Stainless steel	Sirolimus	First
Taxus	Boston Scientific	Stainless steel	Paclitaxel	First
Endeavor	Medtronic	Cobalt–chromium	Zotarolimus	Second
Taxus Liberté	Boston Scientific	Stainless steel	Paclitaxel	Second
Xience	Abbot Vascular	Cobalt–chromium	Everolimus	Second
Promus	Boston Scientific**	Cobalt–chromium	Everolimus	Second

*Cordis is part of the Johnson & Johnson family of companies.
**Promus is a private-labeled Xience coronary stent manufactured by Abbott but distributed by Boston Scientific.

- Everolimus, a derivative of sirolimus, is eluted from Xience (Abbot) and Promus (Boston Scientific) stents. These are exactly the same devices.
- The SPIRIT III trial compared Xience and Taxus Express stents and found significantly less luminal narrowing with the Xience stent. The Xience stent also had significantly fewer major adverse cardiovascular events (MACE) at one year.[24]
- Zotarolimus-eluting stents are represented by Medtronic's Endeavor. When compared with a Cypher stent, the Endeavor stent had more luminal narrowing; however, there was no difference in MACE between the stents.[25]
- The Taxus stent has seen further development in the form of the new Taxus Liberté, which has a lower profile and is easier to deliver to target lesions than the first-generation Taxus Express stent. The polymer and antiproliferative agents are unchanged.
- The current limitation with second-generation DES is data regarding long-term efficacy and safety, especially with regard to late and very late stent thrombosis. Initial results are encouraging and include the recent large Korean ZEST trial,[26] which compared first-generation DES (sirolimus and paclitaxel) with a zotarolimus-eluting stent among all comers with coronary artery disease. The zotarolimus stent had similar MACE compared with the sirolimus stent, but fewer when compared with the paclitaxel stent at 12 months of follow-up. The zotarolimus stent had a lower incidence of repeat procedures than the paclitaxel stent but more than the sirolimus stent. The incidence of stent thrombosis at 1 year was less than 1% with all three DES. The incidence of death and myocardial infarction at 1 year was lowest with the zotarolimus stent.

INDICATIONS FOR CORONARY STENTING

Coronary stenting may be indicated in multiple clinical scenarios. It is important to apply these recommendations to each patient individually and consider all risks and benefits before proceeding with coronary intervention.

Angina

- Angina, or more specifically angina pectoris, is defined as chest discomfort associated with myocardial ischemia without myocardial necrosis. This can be further divided into stable and unstable angina, with the latter being considered an acute coronary syndrome.[27]
- The severity of anginal symptoms is assessed in most circumstances by the Canadian Cardiovascular Society (CCS) class[28] (Table 4). Classes I to III represent stable angina, while class IV usually represents unstable angina.
- Stable angina is chronic and is normally relieved with rest and/or sublingual nitroglycerin.[27]

Table 4 CCS (Canadian Cardiovascular Society) Anginal Classification	
Class I	Ordinary physical activity does not cause angina, such as walking, climbing stairs. Angina occurs with strenuous, rapid, or prolonged exertion at work or recreation.
Class II	Slight limitation of ordinary activity. Angina occurs with climbing more than one flight of stairs.
Class III	Marked limitation of ordinary physical activity. Angina occurs with climbing less than one flight of stairs.
Class IV	Inability to carry on any physical activity without discomfort; angina symptoms may be present at rest.
From Campeau L. Letter: Grading of angina pectoris. *Circulation* 1976;54:522–3. Reprinted with permission from the Canadian Cardiovascular Society.	

- Percutaneous coronary intervention (PCI) is generally considered appropriate in patients with stable angina who have significant coronary disease in one or two major vessels and have one or more of the following[29]:
  - Intermediate- to high-risk findings on noninvasive stress testing
  - Persistent symptoms despite maximal anti-anginal medical therapy
  - High-grade (CCS III and IV) angina regardless of the extent of medical therapy or the severity of findings on noninvasive testing
- Angina may be treated medically with long-acting nitrates, beta blockers, calcium channel blockers, and newer agents such as ranolazine (Ranexa).[30,31]
- Recent trials have compared PCI with medical therapy in stable angina:
  - The COURAGE trial[32] was a randomized study comparing PCI with intensive medical therapy and lifestyle modification in patients with stable coronary disease.
  - After more than 4 years of follow-up, there was no significant difference between the two groups in the rates of the composite endpoint of death, myocardial infarction, and stroke. There was also no difference in the rates of hospitalization for acute coronary syndromes.
  - The PCI group had more relief of angina, although the medical therapy group also had some relief.
  - In patients with stable coronary artery disease, medical therapy is a reasonable alternative to PCI, especially for those with minimal symptoms and no high-risk features.
  - Coronary artery bypass grafting (CABG) is indicated in severe coronary disease affecting multiple vessels (three or more) or the left main coronary artery, as well as potentially in diabetic patients with disease in two or

more vessels.[29] The SYNTAX trial[33] compared multi-vessel drug-eluting stents with PCI (including the left main artery) to CABG in severe coronary artery disease. Patients who received PCI required more repeat revascularization procedures than those in the CABG group, although overall mortality was not significantly different. Patients who underwent CABG had more cerebrovascular events at 1 year of follow-up. CABG remains the standard treatment for severe three-vessel or left main coronary artery disease.

Acute Coronary Syndromes

- Unstable angina, non-ST-elevation myocardial infarction (NSTEMI), and ST-elevation myocardial infarction (STEMI) are classified as acute coronary syndromes.
  - Unstable angina is chest discomfort or anginal equivalent occurring at rest, of new onset (within 1 month) or increased severity, duration, or frequency without evidence of myocardial necrosis (elevated troponin, CK, or CK-MB).
  - NSTEMI is clinically similar to unstable angina, but laboratory testing shows evidence of myocardial necrosis but without ST-segment elevation on an electrocardiogram.
  - STEMI is characterized by a clinical presentation as above, with cardiac enzyme positivity as well as evidence of ST-segment elevation on an electrocardiogram.
- PCI is indicated in high-risk patients with unstable angina/NSTEMI whose coronary stenoses are amenable to intervention (Table 5). The benefit of an early invasive strategy in unstable angina/NSTEMI has been shown in randomized trials as well as meta-analyses.
  - The TACTICS TIMI-18 trial[34] compared coronary angiography within 48 hours to initial conservative

Table 5 Unstable Angina/NSTEMI:
Invasive vs. Conservative Therapy

Preferred Strategy	Patient Characteristics
Invasive	Recurrent angina or ischemia at rest or with low-level activities despite intensive medical therapy
	Elevated cardiac biomarkers
	New or presumable new ST-segment depression
	Signs or symptoms of heart failure or worsening mitral regurgitation
	High-risk findings from noninvasive testing
	Hemodynamic instability
	Sustained ventricular tachycardia
	PCI within 6 months or prior CABG
	High risk score (TIMI, GRACE)
	Reduced left ventricular function
Conservative	Low risk score (TIMI, GRACE)
	Patient or physician preference in absence of high-risk features

From Anderson JL, Adams CD, Antman EM, et al. ACC/AHA 2007 guidelines for the management of patients with unstable angina/non-ST-elevation myocardial infarction. *J Am Coll Cardiol* 2007;50:e1–e157.

therapy (unless continued ischemia was evident) in patients with unstable angina/NSTEMI receiving the IIb/IIIa antagonist tirofiban. There was a significant reduction in MACE in those undergoing early coronary angiography and revascularization.

- A meta-analysis of seven randomized trials of patients with non-ST-elevation acute coronary syndromes randomized to either an early invasive or an initial conservative strategy found a significant decrease in long-term mortality, rates of rehospitalization for unstable angina, and late myocardial infarction.[35]

- In women with unstable angina/NSTEMI and low risk profiles, an initial conservative management strategy can be employed.[36]
- Urgent reperfusion therapy by primary PCI is preferred in STEMI patients with less than 12 hours of symptoms or less than 24 hours when accompanied by persistent ischemia or instability.[29]

PRECATHETERIZATION ASSESSMENT

A thorough assessment is indicated before elective cardiac catheterization and potential PCI. An abbreviated assessment is performed before urgent catheterization. There are few absolute contraindications to cardiac catheterization, but relative contraindications are more numerous.

- As with any procedure, the risks and benefits should be discussed with the patient and consent obtained.
- The medical history should be reviewed, with special attention to prior myocardial infarction, prior cardiac procedures (PCI, CABG, valve repair or replacement) along with any complications, as well as any vascular procedures or diagnoses (abdominal aneurysm with or without repair, lower extremity peripheral arterial disease, etc.). Recent stroke (within 1 month) is a relative contraindication to catheterization and PCI.
- All allergies should be addressed, especially iodinated contrast allergies, which can result in anaphylaxis upon exposure. Prior anesthesia or conscious sedation

history with reactions or complications should also be elucidated.

- Patients with iodinated contrast allergy should be pre-treated with prednisone and antihistamines.

■ Medications should be reviewed and adjusted as appropriate.

- In diabetic patients, dosages of long-acting insulin should be decreased by half the night before the procedure as well as the following morning to avoid periprocedural hypoglycemia while having nothing by mouth.
- Metformin (Glucophage) can result in lactic acidosis after contrast exposure in patients with diabetes and renal insufficiency. This medication should be held before and for at least 48 hours after the procedure.
- Aspirin and clopidogrel dosages do not require adjustment and these medications should be continued.
- In patients with renal insufficiency, hydration with intravenous fluid with or without sodium bicarbonate before and after the procedure has been shown to decrease the incidence of contrast nephropathy.[37] Some studies have shown that the administration of N-acetylcysteine decreases the incidence of contrast nephropathy.[38]

■ Basic laboratory assessment

- A complete blood count is necessary to evaluate for anemia and thrombocytopenia. Acute gastrointestinal bleeding and significant anemia are relative and potentially absolute contraindications to cardiac catheterization.
- A coagulation panel also assesses bleeding risk. In general, the international normalized ratio (INR) should be less than 1.8, but different operators use different

thresholds. Patients receiving warfarin therapy should stop this medication approximately 5 days before the procedure, with an enoxaparin (Lovenox) bridge if indicated.

- A basic metabolic panel assesses renal function and potential electrolyte derangement. Preexisting renal insufficiency predisposes a patient to contrast-induced nephropathy, while electrolyte imbalance may increase the risk of arrhythmia.
- Women of childbearing age should have a pregnancy test before fluoroscopy.

■ Vital signs should be documented. Fever, uncontrolled hypertension, hypotension, and rhythm disturbance increase procedural risk. A focused examination should be performed with careful attention to cardiac/pulmonary auscultation as well as assessment of femoral and distal lower extremity pulses.

■ Patient compliance should also be assessed. Patients undergoing PCI will be prescribed antiplatelet therapy, with the duration of therapy being dictated by the type of stent deployed. Patients with questionable compliance may benefit from BMS placement, as the minimum duration of clopidogrel therapy is only 1 month based on current recommendations versus 1 year for DES. Continued optimal medical therapy without PCI may also be an option for noncompliant patients.

■ Anticipation of scheduled surgical procedures is also important in determining the type of coronary stent that should be used. This is because most surgical procedures require that clopidogrel therapy be held perioperatively. In this situation, a BMS may be preferable to a DES.

STENT DELIVERY

- Coronary stents are delivered to target vessels during cardiac catheterization. Vascular access is most commonly obtained via the right femoral artery, but the left femoral artery as well as brachial and radial approaches may also be used.

- Diagnostic coronary angiography usually precedes coronary intervention, with the left and right coronary arteries being selectively engaged by catheters whose shape and contour enable access to the respective coronary ostia. There are multiple types of catheter shapes and sizes, with aortic and coronary anatomy dictating which is used (for example, anomalous coronary arteries may require a different-shaped catheter to be engaged).

- After engagement of the coronary ostia, iodinated contrast dye is injected into the artery and visualized with the simultaneous use of cine fluoroscopy. A typical coronary angiogram is seen in Figure 2.

- Each major vessel (left main, left anterior descending, left circumflex, and right coronary artery) is ideally evaluated in two separate orthogonal views. This enables stenoses to be adequately visualized and their severity assessed. Lesions are generally considered significant if the vessel is at least 70% stenosed, but the visual determination of lesion severity is operator-dependent.

- In addition to direct observation via angiography, the significance of lesions can be assessed by intravascular ultrasound (IVUS) as well as determination of the fractional flow reserve (FFR).
  - IVUS (Fig. 3) assesses luminal size as well as atherosclerotic plaque burden and morphology via a coronary catheter equipped with an ultrasound transducer. The

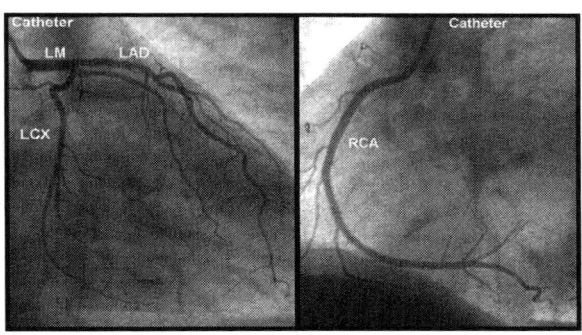

Figure 2 Normal coronary angiogram. LM = left main coronary artery, LAD = left anterior descending coronary artery, LCX = left circumflex coronary artery, RCA = right coronary artery

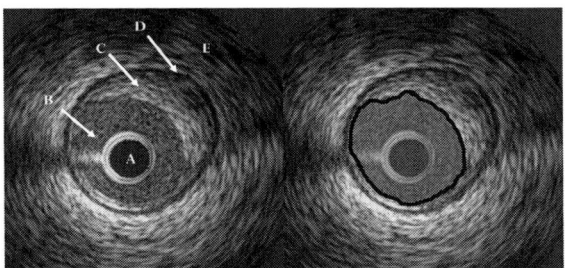

Figure 3 Intracoronary IVUS images. A) IVUS catheter. B) Arterial lumen. C) Atheromatous plaque within the media. D) External elastic membrane, which is the interface between the media and adventitia. E) Adventitia. The right panel highlights the minimal luminal area (MLA) with the circumferential outline representing the interface between the one-cell-layer intima and the beginning of the media.

probe is slowly withdrawn through the vessel in question, providing cross-sectional views. It may also be used to evaluate previously deployed stents—for example, to determine stent strut apposition and the degree of ISR, if present. Various measurements are made, with the most important being the minimal luminal area (MLA). In major coronary arteries (other than the left main), intermediate stenoses with a MLA greater than 3.0 to 4.0 mm2 via IVUS imaging are associated with a low clinical event rate[39,40] and are unlikely to benefit from revascularization. The threshold MLA for a left main stenosis is 6.0 to 7.5 mm2, with revascularization generally recommended below these values.[41,42]

- FFR is a ratio of maximal flow downstream from a coronary stenosis compared with normal upstream flow.[43] Values of 0.75 or less characterize lesions as likely to provoke ischemia with an accuracy greater than 90%.[44] The FAME trial[45] compared angiography-guided PCI with FFR-guided PCI in patients with multivessel coronary disease using a slightly higher FFR significance value of 0.80. Patients in the angiography alone group received DES if a stenosis was deemed significant by the operator, while FFR-guided patients received DES only if the FFR ratio was less than 0.80 across the lesion in question. The FFR-guided PCI patients had significantly fewer events (death, nonfatal myocardial infarction, repeat revascularization) at 1 year, with both groups having similar freedom from angina.

- Once a lesion is determined to be significant and appropriate for PCI, the diagnostic catheter is exchanged for a guide catheter. Guide catheters allow stent delivery systems to be passed to the ostia of the left or right coronary artery.

- Once a guide catheter is in place, a small guide wire is advanced through the catheter into the vessel and across the lesion in question. Multiple guide wires are available, and they vary in terms of stiffness (especially at the tip), strength, as well as hydrophobic versus hydrophilic properties.
- After the guide wire is positioned across the lesion and into the distal aspect of the vessel, balloons for angioplasty as well as stents may be passed over the wire to the

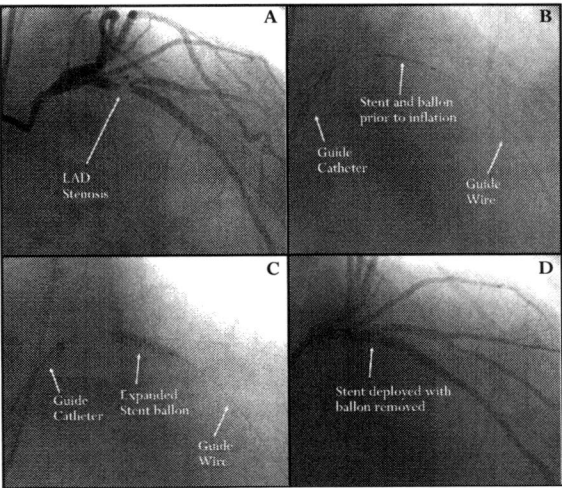

Figure 4 A) Coronary angiogram with a significant stenosis involving the proximal left anterior descending at the takeoff of a large diagonal branch. B) Passage of a stent (mounted on a balloon) over a guide wire positioned across the stenosis. C) Inflation of the balloon, effectively deploying the stent. D) Final result with stent deployed and balloon removed; no residual stenosis.

lesion. Coronary stents are mounted on balloons that, when inflated, deploy the stent. The stent balloon is then deflated, leaving the stent permanently in place (Fig. 4).

- Angioplasty balloons are highly variable, with key characteristics being their length, diameter, and degree of compliance. They also differ with respect to the pressure required for sufficient inflation.
- After stent delivery, the balloon and guide wire are removed. Images are again obtained to ensure a good result as well as to evaluate for signs of vessel injury.

COMPLICATIONS OF CORONARY STENTING

In general, cardiac catheterization and PCI are not considered high-risk procedures. However, complications still occur, necessitating a thorough precatheterization assessment as well as keen attention to detail during and after the procedure. Patient factors such as age, comorbidities, and hemodynamic status, as well as the complexity of the intervention being performed, all play a role in risk determination. Table 6 lists the most common complications of diagnostic catheterization and PCI.

- The most common complication of cardiac catheterization (and thus PCI) is bleeding. This is largely due to arterial access in combination with the likely presence of multiple antithrombotic and antiplatelet agents, which interfere with intrinsic coagulation.
  - A hematoma occurs when blood extravasates into the surrounding tissues; the subcutaneous collection can become quite large and even life-threatening. Most are treated with manual compression and close observation.
  - A pseudoaneurysm is a vascular complication that occurs when a hematoma is in direct communication with the

Table 6 Incidence of Complications Associated with Cardiac Catheterization and PCI

Complication	Incidence (%)
Diagnostic Catheterization[1]	
Death	0.11
Myocardial infarction	0.05
Neurologic	0.07
Arrhythmia	0.38
Contrast-mediated	0.37
Hemodynamic	0.26
Perforation	0.03
PCI[2]	
Death	1.4
Myocardial infarction	0.4
CABG	1.9
Dissection	5.0
Bleeding (Diagnostic + PCI)[3]	
Hematoma (>10 cm)	0.3–1.1
Pseudoaneurysm	0.2–0.5
Retroperitoneal bleed	0.2–0.5
Other major bleeding	0.1–0.4

[1]Noto TJ, Jr., Johnson LW, Krone R, et al. Cardiac catheterization 1990: a report of the Registry of the Society for Cardiac Angiography and Interventions (SCA&I). *Cathet Cardiovasc Diagn* 1991;24:75–83.
[2]Anderson HV, Shaw RE, Brindis RG, et al. A contemporary overview of percutaneous coronary interventions. The American College of Cardiology-National Cardiovascular Data Registry (ACC-NCDR). *J Am Coll Cardiol* 2002;39:1096–103.
[3]Applegate RJ, Sacrinty MT, Kutcher MA, et al. Trends in vascular complications after diagnostic cardiac catheterization and percutaneous coronary intervention via the femoral artery, 1998 to 2007. *JACC Cardiovasc Interv* 2008;1:317–26.

arteriotomy site through a tract, resulting in pulsatile flow. A pseudoaneurysm can often be distinguished from a hematoma by the presence of an audible bruit over the area as well as palpable pulsations. Pseudoaneurysms can be diagnosed via Doppler ultrasound and often require surgical repair or thrombin injection, depending on their size and extent; smaller ones may be treated with compression (ultrasound-guided). Vascular surgery input may be helpful in evaluating a pseudoaneurysm.

- Retroperitoneal bleeding is a particularly serious complication; a high level of suspicion is required for diagnosis. It is commonly associated with an arteriotomy site above the inguinal ligament. Patients may complain of back or abdominal pain after the procedure or may have signs of blood loss, including tachycardia and hypotension. There may be no overt signs of blood loss. Retroperitoneal bleeding may be treated conservatively with blood products, but percutaneous or surgical treatment may be required for hemodynamic instability.

■ Iodinated contrast agents administered during the procedure can have several untoward effects.
  - Contrast-induced nephropathy is usually encountered in patients with pre-existing renal insufficiency. The risk can be reduced by preprocedural hydration as well as administration of N-acetylcysteine, as discussed previously. Treatment is supportive, with hydration and close renal surveillance.
  - Contrast allergy and anaphylaxis are rare. Patients with a known contrast allergy should be pretreated with prednisone and antihistamines. Documented anaphylaxis to a contrast agent is a relative but not an absolute contraindication to cardiac catheterization.

- Cardiovascular complications are associated with increased morbidity as well as mortality.
  - Brief (several seconds) atrial and ventricular arrhythmias during cardiac catheterization can occur due to direct catheter contact with the myocardium (for example, when measuring left ventricular pressure or performing right heart catheterization). More lethal sustained arrhythmias are much less common and may be observed with reperfusion after an intervention on an occluded vessel or in patients with existing conduction system abnormalities or severe left ventricular dysfunction.
  - Injuries to the coronary arteries as well as the aorta are rare but can result in perforation, dissection, or thrombus formation and resultant myocardial infarction. Urgent coronary artery bypass surgery is rarely required in certain situations, depending on the extent and nature of the injury, and in cases of abrupt vessel closure. Although the incidence of emergency CABG has decreased significantly since PCI began, it still carries a significant mortality rate of 10% to 14%.[46]
  - Disruption of aortic plaque through catheter and wire manipulation can result in embolism to the brain, resulting in stroke. Injection of air into the system (air embolus) can also cause stroke or myocardial infarction. Emboli may also pass to the extremities, as evidenced by ischemic digits (normally the toes), or to the kidneys, as evidenced by renal failure, as well as skin changes in the lower extremities (livedo reticularis).
  - Hemodynamic instability may occur, especially in patients who are already in cardiogenic shock and in need of urgent catheterization to re-establish coronary perfusion.

- Complications after stent deployment can be divided into acute (occurring in the catheterization laboratory), subacute (up to 30 days after the procedure), and late (after 30 days). Acute complications, including abrupt closure, vessel dissection, and distal embolization, are usually treated with mechanical or pharmacologic means in the catheterization laboratory. Subacute and late stent thrombosis is a serious complication that may result in complete vessel closure and subsequent myocardial infarction; it can occur with both BMS and DES. Although estimates vary, subacute or late stent thrombosis is generally agreed to occur in 1% to 2% of patients and is often associated with premature discontinuation of dual antiplatelet therapy.[47] ISR is a delayed complication of stent implantation and occurs less frequently with DES. It most often is manifested by angina, but it can present as an acute coronary syndrome.[48]

MEDICAL THERAPY

Medical therapy before, during, and after stent deployment is essential in preventing periprocedural and late complications. The main categories of medications associated with PCI are antiplatelet and antithrombotic agents, in addition to standard medical therapy for patients with known coronary artery disease. Medications associated with coronary stenting as well as their dosing information are listed in Table 7.

- All patients undergoing PCI should be pretreated with aspirin as well as clopidogrel. Significant benefit was shown in the CREDO and PCI-CURE trials in patients undergoing PCI who were pretreated with aspirin and clopidogrel and continued on long-term treatment with both agents for up to 12 months.[49,50] The postprocedure

Table 7 Common Antiplatelet and Antithrombin Medications

Class	Medication	Dosing	
Antiplatelet	Aspirin	Preprocedure:	81–325 mg with 325 mg if aspirin-naïve
		Bare metal stent:	162–325 mg/d x 1 mo, then 75–162 mg/d indefinitely
		Drug-eluting stent:	162–325 mg/d x 3 mo after sirolimus stent
			162–325 mg/d x 6 mo after paclitaxel stent
			75–162 mg/d indefinitely after above
	Clopidogrel (Plavix)	Preprocedure:	300–600 mg PO (600-mg dose if urgent or <6 hrs)
		Bare metal stent:	75 mg/d x 1–12 months
		Drug-eluting stent:	75 mg/d x at least 1 year
	Ticlopidine (Ticlid)	Loading dose:	500 mg PO
		Maint dose:	250 mg PO bid
	Prasugrel (Effient)*	Loading dose:	60 mg PO
		Maint dose:	10 mg PO daily
Glycoprotein IIb/IIIa inhibitor	Abciximab (ReoPro)	Loading dose:	0.25 mg/kg IV
		Maint dose:	0.125 ug/kg/min
		Max dose:	10 ug/min for 12 hrs
	Eptifibatide (Integrilin)	Loading dose†:	180 ug/kg IV bolus
		Maint dose:	2.0 ug/kg/min
		Decrease infusion rate by 50% if CrCl < 50 ml/min.	

(Continued)

Table 7 Continued

Class	Medication	Dosing	
	Tirofiban (Aggrastat)	Loading dose:	0.4 ug/kg/min for 30 min
		Maint dose:	0.1 ug/kg/min
		If CrCl < 30 ml/min, decrease infusion rate by 50%.	
Antithrombin agents	Heparin	PCI:	60–100 units/kg IV with target ACT 250–350
		PCI + IIb/IIIa inhibitor:	50–70 units/kg IV to target ACT 200s
	Enoxaparin (Lovenox)	Loading dose:	30 mg IV bolus
		Maint dose:	1 mg/kg SC q 12 hrs
	Bivalirudin (Angiomax)	During PCI:	0.5–0.75 mg/kg IV bolus, then 1.75 mg/kg/h
	Fondaparinox (Arixtra)	Loading and Maint dose:	2.5 mg SC once daily (additional unfractionated heparin recommended during PCI to prevent catheter thrombosis)

Due to an increased risk of bleeding, Prasugrel (Effient) should not be used in patients with a history of stroke or TIA and should be deferred in patients > 75 years of age unless there is high clinical risk. It may be considered at a reduced dose (5 mg daily) among patients weighing < 60 kg.

[†] A second IV bolus of eptifibatide is often given 10 minutes after the first during PCI.

duration of dual antiplatelet therapy varies depending on the type of stent used.

- Those who are already taking aspirin chronically are given 75 to 325 mg aspirin before PCI.[15] Those who are aspirin-naïve receive 325 mg of aspirin before the procedure.
- An oral loading dose of clopidogrel is also recommended before PCI. If PCI is to be performed urgently, the preferred dose is 600 mg; if PCI is elective or anticipated, a 300-mg dose can be given followed by 75 mg daily until the procedure (300-mg loading dose must be given at least 6 hours before PCI).
- After stent implantation, patients should remain on aspirin (162 to 325 mg) for at least 1 month, with continuation indefinitely at a dose of 81 to 162 mg.
- Clopidogrel (75 mg daily) is continued for at least 1 month after BMS placement, with consideration of therapy for up to 1 year unless there is an increased bleeding risk or other contraindication. For DES, clopidogrel is continued for at least 12 months.[15] Some clinicians will continue clopidogrel longer than the recommended 1-year duration in DES patients in an attempt to decrease the risk of late stent thrombosis, provided clopidogrel continuation does not confer more risk than benefit.
- Ticlopidine, an older thienopyridine, has similar efficacy as clopidogrel but has significantly more hematologic side effects, including anemia, neutropenia, and thrombotic thrombocytopenic purpura.
- Prasugrel is a newer antiplatelet agent that is similar to clopidogrel and ticlopidine but more effectively inhibits the ADP receptor. Compared with clopidogrel in moderate- to high-risk acute coronary syndrome patients

undergoing PCI in the TRITON-TIMI 38 trial, the composite end point of cardiovascular death, nonfatal myocardial infarction, and nonfatal stroke occurred significantly less often in the prasugrel-treated patients at a median duration of therapy of 15 months.[51] However, there was also a significant increase in life-threatening bleeding in the prasugrel-treated patients; this appeared to be confined to the elderly (≥75 years), those with low body weight (<60 kg), and those with a prior history of stroke/transient ischemic attack.

- Glycoprotein IIb/IIIa receptor antagonists such as tirofiban (Aggrastat), eptifibatide (Integrilin), and abciximab (ReoPro) can be given intravenously in conjunction with aspirin and clopidogrel during PCI. Multiple trials have shown the benefit of these medications in acute coronary syndromes; however, many of these studies predated the routine use of clopidogrel. These agents are usually continued for 12 to 18 hours after the procedure, depending on the drug; however, the ideal duration of therapy has recently been called into question, specifically with eptifibatide.[52]

- Antithrombotic medications in the form of heparin (intravenous unfractionated heparin or subcutaneous low-molecular-weight heparin [Lovenox]) or a direct thrombin inhibitor are given to all patients undergoing PCI.

  • For elective PCI, many operators prefer unfractionated heparin because its effects are more easily monitored in the catheterization laboratory (via measurement of the activated clotting time). The short half-life and the ability to reverse the effects of unfractionated heparin with protamine are advantageous in the event of a bleeding complication. The anticoagulant effects of low-molec-ular-weight heparin cannot be monitored as easily; in addition, there is no reversal agent that can be given, and its effects last up to 12 hours after administration.

- Bivalirudin (Angiomax), a direct thrombin inhibitor, is an acceptable alternative to heparin plus a glycoprotein IIb/IIIa inhibitor in elective PCI[53] and acute coronary syndromes.[54,55] This agent is popular in many catheterization laboratories.

- In patients with a heparin allergy or a history of heparin-induced thrombocytopenia, bivalirudin or argatroban (another direct thrombin inhibitor) should be used.

- All patients undergoing coronary stenting should receive standard medications indicated for those with known coronary artery disease. These include statin drugs for effective lipid lowering. In addition, all patients undergoing PCI should be closely followed for aggressive risk factor modification, including blood pressure control in those with hypertension as well as blood glucose control in diabetics. Lifestyle modification is also essential, with diet and exercise counseling.

PERIOPERATIVE MANAGEMENT

About 5% of patients who have received a coronary stent will undergo a noncardiac surgical procedure within the first year after implantation.[56] With millions of individuals undergoing PCI with stenting on an annual basis, the number of patients taking dual antiplatelet therapy in the perioperative period is substantial. Due to the perceived increased risk of surgical bleeding complications, many of these patients are asked to discontinue antiplatelet therapy before surgery, often prematurely with respect to the recommended duration of therapy and without cardiology consultation. This puts patients at increased risk for stent complications, chiefly stent thrombosis, which normally presents as an acute myocardial infarction with significant morbidity and mortality.

- The mechanisms underlying stent thrombosis in the perioperative period, especially around the time of stent implantation, center on the increased thrombogenicity of stents before the formation of a complete endothelium. This combines with the hypercoagulable state after surgery to increase the risk of stent thrombosis.
- Most studies of outcomes in patients with coronary stents undergoing noncardiac surgery address those with BMS. The current ACC/AHA guidelines recommend delaying

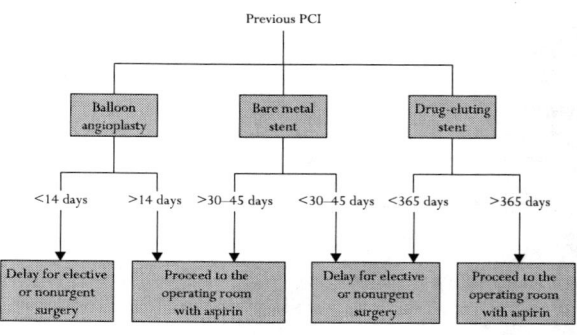

Figure 5 Management of patients with prior PCI who require noncardiac surgery based on time since PCI. (Reprinted from Fleisher LA, Beckman JA, Brown KA, et al. ACC/AHA guidelines on perioperative cardiovascular evaluation and care for noncardiac surgery. *Circulation* 2007;116:1971–96. Copyright © 2007, American Heart Association, Inc. With permission from Wolters Kluwer Health.)

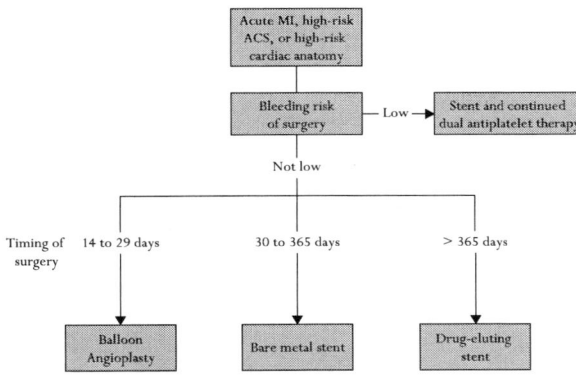

Figure 6 Treatment for patients requiring PCI who may need subsequent surgery. (Reprinted from Fleisher LA, Beckman JA, Brown KA, et al. ACC/AHA guidelines on perioperative cardiovascular evaluation and care for noncardiac surgery. *Circulation* 2007;116:1971–96. Copyright © 2007, American Heart Association, Inc. With permission from Wolters Kluwer Health.)

noncardiac surgery for 4 to 6 weeks after BMS placement.[57] Algorithms for patients with previous stents who require noncardiac surgery as well as for patients in whom PCI may be required before surgery are shown in Figures 5 and 6, respectively. However, preoperative stress testing with potential revascularization remains controversial.[58,59]

- Multiple studies have documented an increased risk of periprocedural death or myocardial infarction when surgery is performed within 2 to 3 weeks after BMS implantation.[60,61] However, this risk may persist for as long as 6 weeks after stent implantation.[62] In a significant proportion of the patients in these studies, aspirin and/or thienopyridine treatment was discontinued before surgery, although in many patients periprocedural antiplatelet therapy was continued.

- Data regarding DES and noncardiac surgery are limited, but similar results are shown with premature discontinuation of antiplatelet therapy.
  - Analysis of the PREMIER registry of patients receiving DES noted a nine-fold increase in mortality in patients who discontinued antiplatelet therapy during the first 11 months after implantation.[63]
  - A large study of DES patients noted that premature discontinuation of dual antiplatelet therapy (within 6 months of implantation) was the most important predictor of stent thrombosis, with thrombosis occurring in 29% of patients who stopped aspirin and clopidogrel prematurely. Patients who had stent thrombosis had a case fatality rate of 45%.[19]
- Dual antiplatelet therapy is problematic for surgical procedures due to the inherent potential for bleeding complications. However, the risk of continuation of therapy must be weighed against the risk of stent thrombosis from cessation. Clopidogrel and ticlopidine irreversibly inhibit platelets for about 5 days until new platelets can be produced; therefore, these medications are often held for 5 to 10 days preoperatively if required.
- Proposed mechanisms for reducing periprocedural stent thrombosis include the following[23,64]
  - Before stent implantation, the need for dual antiplatelet therapy should be discussed. In patients not expected to comply, DES placement should be avoided.
  - In patients likely to undergo invasive or surgical procedures in the next 12 months who are deemed likely to

benefit from revascularization, placement of a BMS or performance of balloon angioplasty should be considered instead of DES placement.

- Patients should be thoroughly educated about why dual antiplatelet therapy is being prescribed and the extreme risks of premature discontinuation.
- Patients should be instructed to contact their cardiologist before stopping any antiplatelet therapy for any reason.
- Providers performing invasive or surgical procedures who are concerned about bleeding complications should also be familiar with the risks of discontinuation of antiplatelet therapy.
- Elective procedures with an increased risk of bleeding should be deferred until patients have completed the recommended course of antiplatelet therapy.
- Patients with DES who are undergoing procedures that require the discontinuation of thienopyridine therapy should continue aspirin if possible. Thienopyridine therapy should be resumed as soon as possible after the procedure.
- Other options are available, but there are few data supporting these methods. Some physicians have used bridging therapy with either intravenous glycoprotein IIb/IIIa inhibitors or antithrombotic agents in high-risk patients in the interval between clopidogrel discontinuation and surgery.

STENT SURVEILLANCE

After stent implantation, patients are usually observed in the hospital overnight with telemetry monitoring and serial electrocardiograms; however, this practice has recently been called into question in low-risk patients.[65] There should be a low threshold for repeat catheterization in patients with anginal symptoms and objective evidence of ischemia in the immediate postprocedure period.

- After stent implant and observation for periprocedural complications, patients are generally followed by a cardiologist to assess for signs or symptoms of angina or anginal equivalent, which could indicate worsening native coronary artery disease or restenosis of previously placed stents.
- Current guidelines do not recommend noninvasive testing in asymptomatic individuals after PCI unless there was incomplete revascularization at the initial procedure.[66]
- In post-PCI patients with worsening symptoms, further testing via invasive or noninvasive means is necessary. Proceeding directly to repeat heart catheterization or performing a noninvasive stress test is operator-dependent, taking into account the patient's burden of disease, severity of symptoms, and other comorbidities. In general, repeat catheterization is recommended when PCI occurred in the previous 6 months, since this is the time frame when restenosis is most likely to occur. Any patient suspected of having acute coronary syndrome should undergo invasive evaluation.
- Patients should also be followed for adherence to anti-platelet therapy for the recommended treatment period. Other medical comorbidities should be addressed and optimized, including blood pressure, lipid profiles, and glycemic control in diabetic patients. Diet and exercise management are also essential in further reducing the risk for cardiac events. Both CABG and PCI patients can benefit from cardiac rehabilitation.[67]

FUTURE DEVELOPMENTS

The field of interventional cardiology is characterized by rapid change and constantly evolving technology. Developments occur so quickly that some devices become obsolete soon after release. There are many new iterations of stent technology under development, attempting to address the limitations of currently available devices. There are new developments in stent platforms and delivery technology and new approaches to challenging coronary anatomy. This section will address the improvements in PCI under development.

- The number of next-generation stents under investigation is substantial (see Appendix). They all attempt to inhibit the restenotic process while addressing the safety concerns of the DES currently available. Strategies include fully bioabsorbable polymer and stent platforms, biodegradable polymer, non-polymer-coated platforms with drug delivery, the combination of antiproliferative and antithrombotic/antiplatelet agents, nanotechnology, and pro-healing technology. A sampling of newer-generation stents is presented below.
  - The Bioabsorbable Vascular Solutions (BVS) poly-L-lactic acid stent platform is coated with an everolimus-containing polylactic acid polymer. The ABSORB study evaluated this fully bioabsorbable device in 30 patients. At 2 year follow-up there were no deaths, target lesion revascularizations (TLR), or stent thromboses and a single non-ST-segment myocardial infarction. Multiple imaging modalities suggested a low late loss and percent diameter stenosis.[68]
  - The ISAR-TEST 3 trial compared three sirolimus-eluting stents with different polymer strategies, which included Cypher (permanent polymer), a biodegradable

polymer stent, and a polymer-free device. Late loss was significantly higher with the polymer-free stent compared with the permanent or biodegradable polymer.[69]

- The ISAR-TEST-4 trial compared the same sirolimus-eluting biodegradable polymer stent to the permanent polymer Cypher and Xience stents. At 1 year the biodegradable polymer stent was non-inferior to Cypher and Xience for the clinical end points of death, myocardial infarction, and TLR. The stent thrombosis rate was not different.[70]

- MAHOROBA is a cobalt–chromium alloy stent employing a bioabsorbable poly-D,L-lactide-co-glycolide (PLGA) coating eluting tacrolimus. This device was studied in 47 patients. The 4-month late loss was 0.99 ± 0.46 mm and the 6-month clinical event rate included 2 myocardial infarctions and 11 ischemia-driven repeat interventions.[71]

- The non-polymer-based Vestasync stent has a stainless steel platform and nanothin microporous hydroxyapatite polymer-free surface impregnated with the antiproliferative agent sirolimus. In a first-in-man study Vestasync yielded acceptable late loss at 4 months (0.30 ± 0.25 mm) and no adverse events at 6 months.[72]

- One-year results were recently published for the Catania stent in the ATLANTA trial, a first-in-man evaluation of a cobalt–chromium stent coated with an inorganic nanothin surface of Polyzene-F. Polyzene-F has bacterial resistance and anti-inflammatory properties and inhibits platelet activation and neointimal hyperplasia. In 55 patients, late loss at 6 months was 0.60 ± 0.48 mm. The 12-month clinically driven rate of TLR was 3.6%. There were no deaths, myocardial infarctions, or stent thromboses. Importantly, in an analysis of stent strut coverage by optical coherence tomography, 99.5% of all stent struts were covered.[73]

- A novel concept being developed is the Custom NX stent (formerly Xtent) system. This platform can treat lesions up to 60 mm long with 6-mm interdigitated stent segments mounted on a single device. One or more segments can be delivered at a time, allowing treatment of different lengths or multiple lesions. The delivery balloon is resizable, avoiding the need for a second postdilatation balloon. The stent is cobalt–chromium alloy with a biodegradable polymer on the abluminal surface containing the sirolimus derivative Biolimus A9. In the CUSTOM II trial 100 patients were implanted for either long lesions or two different lesions. The MACE rate at 1 year was 9%. The TLR rate was 4%, with one in-hospital stent thrombosis. Late loss was 0.31 ± 0.31 mm.[74] The CUSTOM IV and CUSTOM IV Angio trials have recently been approved by the Food and Drug Administration.

- The Genous stent stainless steel platform is coated with an immobilized monoclonal antibody directed at surface antigens of endothelial progenitor cells. This theoretically promotes early healing while reducing the risk of hypersensitivity or inflammation from polymer or drug elution so that a shorter duration of antiplatelet therapy could be used. TRIAS-HR showed favorable results in 98 Genous compared to 95 Taxus patients with a lower myocardial infarction but higher TLR rate.[75] The E-Healing registry has reported on 1,640 of 5,000 patients. TLR at 12 months was 5.4%, with one stent thrombosis, using only 30 days of dual antiplatelet therapy.[76] In a 100-patient trial compared to a cobalt–chromium stent in STEMI, late stent thrombosis was increased in Genous patients (6%) and TLR at 6 months was higher (14% vs. 4%, $p = 0.04$).[77] Therefore, this technology remains unproven.

- The percutaneous treatment of bifurcation disease remains challenging. Overall the literature supports a strategy of provisional side branch stenting when approaching bifurcations. The concept is to address the disease in the main vessel and treat the side branch only if complicated by slow flow, significant dissection, or abrupt closure. There are still limitations such as maintaining side branch access, difficulty in side branch rewiring due to main vessel stent jailing, main vessel stent distortion with treatment of a side branch, and incomplete scaffolding at the ostium of the side branch. There are 11 dedicated side branch devices under development, with several strategies being employed.[78]

  - Several devices use the approach of a BMS (stainless steel or cobalt–chromium) incorporating various configurations of side branch access and a one- or two-wire and one- or two-balloon delivery system. These include the Abbott Fontier (Abbott Vascular Devices, Redwood, CA), Invatec Twin-Rail (Invatec S.R.L., Italy), AST SLK-View (Advanced Stent Technologies, CA), Minvasys Nile Croco (Minvasys, France), TriReme Antares SAS (TriReme Medical Inc., CA), Tryton (Tryton Medical, NC), and Y-Med Sidekick (Y-Med, Inc., CA).

  - The Petal (Boston Scientific, MA) and Devax Axxess Plus (Devax, CA) are devices designed to treat bifurcation disease using a drug-eluting platform. The Taxus Petal stent is undergoing clinical investigation.

- The Stentys (Stentys S.A.S., France) design uses a polymer-coated nitinol self-expanding stent with paclitaxel elution. It has the unique feature of balloon-facilitated strut disconnection at the point of the side branch. The disconnected struts then scaffold the side branch ostium.
- Initial treatment of a side branch ostium with the trumpet-shaped self-expanding nitinol Cappella Sideguard (Capella Inc., Ireland) allows standard stenting of the main vessel using the device of choice. A second-generation drug-eluting version is planned.

- Historically, ablative devices were used in an attempt to reduce the ischemic complications of PCI. Several approaches were developed, including directional coronary atherectomy, Excimer laser coronary angioplasty, transluminal rotational atherectomy, transluminal extraction coronary atherectomy, holmium laser, and cutting balloon atherotomy. These techniques had in common the concept of plaque remodeling in an effort to optimize acute results and lower intimal injury and restenosis risk. Most clinical trials were small and underpowered and left unanswered questions. A 2004 meta-analysis of 9,222 patients suggested no angiographic benefit with these devices and further no improvement in clinical outcomes.[79] Currently these technologies are not used as stand-alone therapy. Rotational atherectomy is used with calcified anatomy to facilitate stent placement. Laser atherectomy may be used for ISR, chronic total occlusions, saphenous vein grafts containing thrombus, and acute coronary syndromes.[80]

- The Diamondback 360 Orbital Atherectomy System (CSI, MN) and the Jetstream G2 NXT (Pathway Medical Technologies, WA) are atherectomy devices approved for use in the peripheral vascular circulation. Both technologies are being explored for possible use in the coronary circulation.

PATIENT AND PROVIDER RESOURCES

Organizations

American Heart Association (AHA): www.americanheart.org, www.hearthub.org

American College of Cardiology (ACC): www.acc.org, www.cardiosource.com

AHA/ACC guidelines: www.americanheart.org/presenter. jhtml?identifier=3004542

European Society of Cardiology (ESC): www.escardio.org

ESC guidelines: www.escardio.org/guidelines-surveys/ esc-guidelines/Pages/GuidelinesList.aspx

Society of Cardiovascular Angiography and Interventions: www.scai.org

Transcatheter Therapeutics: www.tctmd.com

Cardiovascular Research Technologies: www.crtonline.org

Industry

Abbott (Multi-link Vision and Xience stents): www.abbott. com, www.abbottvascular.com

Boston Scientific (Taxus, Taxus Liberté, Taxus Express, Promus stents): www.stent.com, www.taxus-stent.com, www.bostonscientific.com

Cordis (Cypher stents): www.cordis.com, www.cypherstent.com

Medtronic (Driver and Endeavor stents): www.medtronic. com, www.endeavorstent.com

Pharmaceuticals

Clopidogrel (Plavix)—Bristol Myers Squibb and Sanofi-Aventis: www.plavix.com, www.bms.com, www.sanofi-aventis.com

Prasugrel (Effient)—Eli Lilly: www.effient.com, www.lilly.com

Eptifibatide (Integrilin)—Millennium Pharmaceuticals: www.integrilin.com, www.mlnm.com

Abciximab (ReoPro)—Eli Lilly, Centocor Ortho Biotech: www.reopro.com

Miscellaneous/General Information

www.cardiologytoday.com

www.heartsite.com

www.cardiologysite.com

www.theheart.org

www.angioplasty.org

REFERENCES

1. Gruntzig AR, Senning A, Siegenthaler WE. Nonoperative dilatation of coronary artery stenosis: percutaneous transluminal coronary angioplasty. *N Engl J Med* 1979;301:61–8.
2. Ten Berg JM, Gin MTJ, Ernst SMPH, et al. Ten-year follow-up of percutaneous transluminal coronary angioplasty for proximal left anterior descending coronary artery stenosis in 351 patients. *J Am Coll Cardiol* 1996;28(1):82–8.

3. Sigwart U, Puel J, Mirkovitch V, et al. Intravascular stents to prevent occlusion and restenosis after transluminal angioplasty. *N Engl J Med* 1987;7:450–7.

4. Roubin GS, Cannon AD, Agrawal SK, et al. Intracoronary stenting for acute and threatened vessel closure complicating percutaneous transluminal coronary angioplasty. *Circulation* 1992;85:916–27.

5. Serruys PW, de Jaegere P, Macaya C, et al. A randomized comparison of balloon expandable stent implantation with balloon angioplasty in patients with coronary artery disease. *N Engl J Med* 1994;331:489–95.

6. Palmaz JC, Sibbitt RR, Reuter SR, et al. Expandable intraluminal graft: a preliminary study: work in progress. *Radiology* 1985;156:73–7.

7. Serruys PW, Emanuelsson H, van der Giessen W, et al. Heparin-coated Palmaz-Schatz stents in human coronary arteries. Early outcome of the Benestent-II pilot study. *Circulation* 1996; 93(3):412–22.

8. Babapulle MN, Joseph L, Belisle P, et al. A hierarchical Bayesian meta-analysis of randomized clinical trials of drug eluting stents. *Lancet* 2004;363:583–91.

9. Bavry AA, Kumbhani DJ, Helton TJ, et al. Late thrombosis of drug-eluting stents; a meta-analysis of randomized clinical trials. *Am J Med* 2006;119:1056–61.

10. Qasim A, Cosgrave J, Latib A, et al. Long term follow-up of drug-eluting stents when inserted for on and off-label indications. *Am J Cardiol* 2007;100(11):1619–24.

11. Chhatriwalla AK, Bhatt DL. Should dual anti-platelet therapy after drug-eluting stents be continued for more than 1 year? *Circ Cardiovasc Intevent* 2008;1:217–25.

12. Cutlip DE, Baim DS, Ho KK, et al. Stent thrombosis in the modern era: a pooled analysis of multi-center coronary stent clinical trials. *Circulation* 2001;103:1967–71.

13. Lau K W, Mak K H, Hung JS, et al. Clinical impact of stent construction and design in percutaneous coronary intervention. *Am Heart J* 2004;147:764–73.

14. Fischman DL, Leon MB, Baim DS, et al. A randomized comparison of coronary-stent placement and balloon angioplasty in the treatment of coronary artery disease. Stent Restenosis Study Investigators. *N Engl J Med* 1994;331:496–501.

15. King SB 3rd, Smith SC Jr., Hirshfeld JW Jr., et al. 2007 Focused Update of the ACC/AHA/SCAI 2005 Guideline Update for Percutaneous Coronary Intervention: a report of the American College of Cardiology/American Heart Association Task Force on Practice Guidelines: 2007 Writing Group to Review New Evidence and Update the ACC/AHA/SCAI 2005 Guideline Update for Percutaneous Coronary Intervention, Writing on Behalf of the 2005 Writing Committee. *Circulation* 2008;117:261–95.

16. Stone GW, Ellis SG, Cox DA, et al. A polymer-based, paclitaxel-eluting stent in patients with coronary artery disease. *N Engl J Med* 2004;350:221–31.

17. Moses JW, Leon MB, Popma JJ, et al. Sirolimus-eluting stents versus standard stents in patients with stenosis in a native coronary artery. *N Engl J Med* 2003;349:1315–23.

18. McFadden EP, Stabile E, Regar E, et al. Late thrombosis in drug-eluting coronary stents after discontinuation of antiplatelet therapy. *Lancet* 2004;364:1519–21.

19. Iakovou I, Schmidt T, Bonizzoni E, et al. Incidence, predictors, and outcome of thrombosis after successful implantation of drug-eluting stents. *JAMA* 2005;293:2126–30.

20. Roukoz H, Bavry AA, Sarkees ML, et al. Comprehensive meta-analysis on drug-eluting stents versus bare-metal stents during extended follow-up. *Am J Med* 2009;122:581 e1–10.

21. Stone GW, Moses JW, Ellis SG, et al. Safety and efficacy of sirolimus- and paclitaxel-eluting coronary stents. *N Engl J Med* 2007;356:998–1008.

22. Kastrati A, Mehilli J, Pache J, et al. Analysis of 14 trials comparing sirolimus-eluting stents with bare-metal stents. *N Engl J Med* 2007;356:1030–9.

23. Grines CL, Bonow RO, Casey DE Jr., et al. Prevention of premature discontinuation of dual antiplatelet therapy in patients with coronary artery stents: a science advisory from the American Heart Association, American College of Cardiology, Society for Cardiovascular Angiography and Interventions, American College of Surgeons, and American Dental Association, with representation from the American College of Physicians. *J Am Coll Cardiol* 2007;49:734–9.

24. Stone GW, Midei M, Newman W, et al. Comparison of an everolimus-eluting stent and a paclitaxel-eluting stent in patients with coronary artery disease: a randomized trial. *JAMA* 2008;299:1903–13.

25. Kandzari DE, Leon MB, Popma JJ, et al. Comparison of zotarolimus-eluting and sirolimus-eluting stents in patients with native coronary artery disease: a randomized controlled trial. *J Am Coll Cardiol* 2006;48:2440–7.

26. Park S-J. Comparison of sirolimus and paclitaxel-eluting stents versus zotarolimus-eluting stents in real world practice: the ZEST randomized controlled trial. Presented at ACC.09/i2. Orlando, FL, 2009.

27. Morrow DA, Gersh BJ, Braunwald E. Chronic coronary artery disease. In: Zipes DP, Libby P, Bonow RO, Braunwald E, eds. *Braunwald's heart disease: a textbook of cardiovascular medicine.* 7 ed. Philadelphia: Saunders, 2005:1281–308.

28. Campeau L. Letter: Grading of angina pectoris. *Circulation* 1976;54:522–3.

29. Patel MR, Dehmer GJ, Hirshfeld JW, et al. ACCF/SCAI/STS/AATS/AHA/ASNC 2009 Appropriateness Criteria for Coronary Revascularization: a report by the American College

of Cardiology Foundation Appropriateness Criteria Task Force, Society for Cardiovascular Angiography and Interventions, Society of Thoracic Surgeons, American Association for Thoracic Surgery, American Heart Association, and the American Society of Nuclear Cardiology Endorsed by the American Society of Echocardiography, the Heart Failure Society of America, and the Society of Cardiovascular Computed Tomography. *J Am Coll Cardiol* 2009;53:530–53.

30. Abrams J. Clinical practice. Chronic stable angina. *N Engl J Med* 2005;352:2524–33.

31. Wilson SR, Scirica BM, Braunwald E, et al. Efficacy of ranolazine in patients with chronic angina observations from the randomized, double-blind, placebo-controlled MERLIN-TIMI (Metabolic Efficiency With Ranolazine for Less Ischemia in Non-ST-Segment Elevation Acute Coronary Syndromes) 36 Trial. *J Am Coll Cardiol* 2009;53:1510–6.

32. Boden WE, O'Rourke RA, Teo KK, et al. Optimal medical therapy with or without PCI for stable coronary disease. *N Engl J Med* 2007;356:1503–16.

33. Serruys PW, Morice MC, Kappetein AP, et al. Percutaneous coronary intervention versus coronary-artery bypass grafting for severe coronary artery disease. *N Engl J Med* 2009; 360:961–72.

34. Cannon CP, Weintraub WS, Demopoulos LA, et al. Comparison of early invasive and conservative strategies in patients with unstable coronary syndromes treated with the glycoprotein IIb/IIIa inhibitor tirofiban. *N Engl J Med* 2001; 344:1879–87.

35. Bavry AA, Kumbhani DJ, Rassi AN, et al. Benefit of early invasive therapy in acute coronary syndromes: a meta-analysis of contemporary randomized clinical trials. *J Am Coll Cardiol* 2006;48:1319–25.

36. Anderson JL, Adams CD, Antman EM, et al. ACC/AHA 2007 guidelines for the management of patients with unstable angina/non-ST-elevation myocardial infarction: a report of the American College of Cardiology/American Heart Association Task Force on Practice Guidelines (Writing Committee to Revise the 2002 Guidelines for the Management of Patients With Unstable Angina/Non-ST-Elevation Myocardial Infarction) developed in collaboration with the American College of Emergency Physicians, the Society for Cardiovascular Angiography and Interventions, and the Society of Thoracic Surgeons endorsed by the American Association of Cardiovascular and Pulmonary Rehabilitation and the Society for Academic Emergency Medicine. *J Am Coll Cardiol* 2007;50:e1-e157.

37. Solomon R, Werner C, Mann D, Silva P. Effects of saline, mannitol, and furosemide to prevent decreases in renal function induced by radiocontrast agents. *New Engl J Med* 1994;331:1416–20.

38. Kelly AM, Dwamena B, Cronin P, et al. Meta-analysis: effectiveness of drugs for preventing contrast-induced nephropathy. *Ann Intern Med* 2008;148:284–94.

39. Abizaid AS, Mintz GS, Mehran R, et al. Long-term follow-up after percutaneous transluminal coronary angioplasty was not performed based on intravascular ultrasound findings: importance of lumen dimensions. *Circulation* 1999;100:256–61.

40. Takagi A, Tsurumi Y, Ishii Y, et al. Clinical potential of intravascular ultrasound for physiological assessment of coronary stenosis: relationship between quantitative ultrasound tomography and pressure-derived fractional flow reserve. *Circulation* 1999;100:250–5.

41. Fassa AA, Wagatsuma K, Higano ST, et al. Intravascular ultrasound-guided treatment for angiographically indetermi-

nate left main coronary artery disease: a long-term follow-up study. *J Am Coll Cardiol* 2005;45:204–11.

42. Jasti V, Ivan E, Yalamanchili V, et al. Correlations between fractional flow reserve and intravascular ultrasound in patients with an ambiguous left main coronary artery stenosis. *Circulation* 2004;110:2831–6.

43. Pijls NH, De Bruyne B, Peels K, et al. Measurement of fractional flow reserve to assess the functional severity of coronary-artery stenoses. *N Engl J Med* 1996;334:1703–8.

44. Pijls NH, Van Gelder B, Van der Voort P, et al. Fractional flow reserve. A useful index to evaluate the influence of an epicardial coronary stenosis on myocardial blood flow. *Circulation* 1995;92:3183–93.

45. Tonino PA, De Bruyne B, Pijls NH, et al. Fractional flow reserve versus angiography for guiding percutaneous coronary intervention. *N Engl J Med* 2009;360:213–24.

46. Yang EH, Gumina RJ, Lennon RJ, et al. Emergency coronary artery bypass surgery for percutaneous coronary interventions: changes in the incidence, clinical characteristics, and indications from 1979 to 2003. *J Am Coll Cardiol* 2005;46:2010–12.

47. Aoki J, Lansky AJ, Mehran R, et al. Early stent thrombosis in patients with acute coronary syndromes treated with drug-eluting and bare metal stents: the Acute Catheterization and Urgent Intervention Triage Strategy trial. *Circulation* 2009;119:687–98.

48. Chen MS, John JM, Chew DP, et al. Bare metal stent restenosis is not a benign clinical entity. *Am Heart J* 2006;151:1260–4.

49. Steinhubl SR, Berger PB, Mann JT 3rd, et al. Early and sustained dual oral antiplatelet therapy following percutaneous coronary intervention: a randomized controlled trial. *JAMA* 2002;288:2411–20.

50. Mehta SR, Yusuf S, Peters RJ, et al. Effects of pretreatment with clopidogrel and aspirin followed by long-term therapy in

patients undergoing percutaneous coronary intervention: the PCI-CURE study. *Lancet* 2001;358:527–33.

51. Wiviott SD, Braunwald E, McCabe CH, et al. Prasugrel versus clopidogrel in patients with acute coronary syndromes. *N Engl J Med* 2007;357:2001–15.

52. Fung AY, Saw J, Starovoytov A, et al. Abbreviated infusion of eptifibatide after successful coronary intervention. The BRIEF-PCI (Brief Infusion of Eptifibatide Following Percutaneous Coronary Intervention) randomized trial. *J Am Coll Cardiol* 2009;53:837–45.

53. Lincoff AM, Bittl JA, Harrington RA, et al. Bivalirudin and provisional glycoprotein IIb/IIIa blockade compared with heparin and planned glycoprotein IIb/IIIa blockade during percutaneous coronary intervention: REPLACE-2 randomized trial. *JAMA* 2003;289:853–63.

54. Stone GW, McLaurin BT, Cox DA, et al. Bivalirudin for patients with acute coronary syndromes. *N Engl J Med* 2006;355:2203–16.

55. Stone GW, Witzenbichler B, Guagliumi G, et al. Bivalirudin during primary PCI in acute myocardial infarction. *N Engl J Med* 2008;358:2218–30.

56. Schouten O, Bax JJ, Poldermans D, et al. Management of patients with cardiac stents undergoing noncardiac surgery. *Curr Opin Anaesthesiol* 2007;20:274–8.

57. Fleisher LA, Beckman JA, Brown KA, et al. ACC/AHA guidelines on perioperative cardiovascular evaluation and care for noncardiac surgery. *Circulation* 2007;116:1971–96.

58. McFalls EO, Ward HB, Moritz TE, et al. Coronary-artery revascularization before elective major vascular surgery. *N Engl J Med* 2004;351:2795–804.

59. Kaluza GL, Joseph J, Lee JR, et al. Catastrophic outcomes of noncardiac surgery soon after coronary stenting. *J Am Coll Cardiol* 2000;34:1288–94.

60. Leibowitz D, Cohen M, Planer D, et al. Comparison of cardiovascular risk of noncardiac surgery following coronary angioplasty with versus without stenting. *Am J Cardiol* 2006;97:1188–91.

61. Sharma AK, Ajani AE, Hamwi SM, et al. Major noncardiac surgery following coronary stenting: when is it safe to operate? *Catheter Cardiovasc Interv* 2004;63:141–5.

62. Wilson WH, Fasseas P, Orford JL, et al. Clinical outcomes of patients undergoing noncardiac surgery in the two months following coronary stenting. *J Am Coll Cardiol* 2003;42:234–40.

63. Spertus JA, Kettelkamp R, Vance C, et al. Prevalence, predictors, and outcomes of premature discontinuation of thienopyridine therapy after drug eluting stent placement: results from the PREMIER registry. *Circulation* 2006;113:2803–9.

64. Bavry AA, Bhatt DL. Appropriate use of drug-eluting stents: balancing the reduction in restenosis with the concern of late thrombosis. *Lancet* 2008;371:2134–43.

65. Heyde GA, Koch KT, Robbert JDW, et al. Randomized trial comparing same-day discharge with overnight hospital stay after PCI: results of the Elective PCI in Outpatient Study (EPOS). *Circulation* 2007;115:2299–306.

66. Hendel RC, Berman DS, Di Carli MF, et al. 2009 appropriate use criteria for cardiac radionucleotide imaging. *Circulation* 2009;119:e561–87.

67. Dendale P, Berger J, Hansen D, et al. Cardiac rehabilitation reduces the rate of major adverse cardiac events after percutaneous coronary intervention. *Eur J Cardiovasc Nurs* 2005;4:113–6.

68. Serruys PW, Ormiston JA, Onuma Y, et al. A bioabsorbable everolimus-eluting coronary stent system (ABSORB): 2-year outcomes and results from multiple imaging methods. *Lancet* 2009 Mar 14;373:897–910.

69. Mehilli J, Byrne RA, Wieczorek A, et al. Randomized trial of three rapamycin-eluting stents with different coating

strategies for reduction of coronary restenosis. *Eur Heart J* 2008;29:1975–82.

70. Byrne RA, Kastrati A, Kufner S, et al. Randomized, non-inferiority trial of three limus agent-eluting stents with different polymer coatings: the Intracoronary Stenting and Angiographic Results: Test Efficacy of 3 Limus-Eluting Stents (ISAR-TEST-4) Trial. *Eur Heart J* 2009 Aug 30 (Epub ahead of print)

71. Onuma Y, Serruys P, den Heijer P, et al. MAHAROBA, first-in-man study: 6-month results of a biodegradable polymer sustained release tacrolimus-eluting stent in *de novo* coronary stenoses. *Eur Heart J* 2009:30:1477–85.

72. Costa JR, Abizaid A, Costa R, et al. Preliminary results of the hydroxyapatite nonpolymer-based sirolimus-eluting stent for the treatment of single de novo coronary lesions. A first-in-human analysis of a third-generation drug-eluting stent system. *J Am Coll Cardiol Interv* 2008;1:545–51.

73. Tamburino C, La Manna A, Di Salvo ME, et al. First-in-man 1-year clinical outcomes of the Catania Coronary Stent System with nanothin Polyzene-F in de novo native coronary artery lesions. The ATLANTA (Assessment of the LAtest Non-Thrombogenic Angioplasty stent) Trial. *J Am Coll Cardiol Interv* 2009;2:197–204.

74. Stella PR, Mueller R, Pavlakis G, et al. One year results of a new in situ length-adjustable stent platform with a biodegradable biolimus A9 eluting polymer: results of the CUSTOM-II trial. *Eurointervention* 2008 Aug;4(2):200–7.

75. The TRIAS-HR pilot study. Presented by Dr. Robertt de Winter at Transcatheter Cardiovascular Therapeutics (TCT) Conference, Washington, DC, October 2007.

76. Silber S, de Winter R, Grisold M, et al. Second- and Third-Generation Drug-Eluting Stent Technology, Abstract 6000:

Clinical outcome for the endothelial progenitor cells capturing Genous Stent: first results of the 1-year follow-up in 5000 Patients. *Circulation* 2008;118:S1043.

77. A randomized comparison of Genous stent versus chromium-cobalt stent for treatment of ST-elevation myocardial infarction: a 6-Month clinical, angiographic, and IVUS follow-up: GENIUS-STEMI trial. Presented by Dr. Pavel Cervinka at ACC.09/i2, Orlando, FL, March 2009.

78. Sheiban I, Omede P, Biondi-Zoccai, G, et al. Update on dedicated bifurcation stents. *J Interven Cardiol* 2009;22:150—5.

79. Bittl JA, Chew DP, Topol EJ, et al. Meta-analysis of randomized trials of percutaneous transluminal angioplasty versus atherectomy, cutting balloon atherotomy, or laser angioplasty. *J Am Coll Cardiol* 2004;43:936—42.

80. Topaz O, Ebersole D, Das T, et al. Excimer laser angioplasty in acute myocardial infarction (the CARMEL multicenter trial). *Am J Cardiol* 2004;93(6):694—701.

APPENDIX

Company	Product Name	Notes	Polymer Type	Drug	Status US	Status OUS
Aachen Resonance	ARTAX		No polymer	Paclitaxel	NA	CE Mark approval gained
Aachen Resonance	VITA Stent		Durable	Tretinoin		CE Mark approval gained
Abbott	PathFinder	Bifurcation lesions	Durable	Everolimus	Preclinicals under way	Preclinicals under way
Abbott	Xience		Durable	Everolimus	On the market	CE Mark approval gained
Abbott	Xience NANO	Small vessel 2.25 mm	Durable	Everolimus	US clinical trial under way	CE Mark approval gained
Abbott	Xience PRIME		Durable	Everolimus	US clinical trial under way	CE Mark approval gained
Abbott	Bioabsorbable stent	Bioabsorbable stent	Bioabsorbable	Everolimus		Feasibility study under way
Alvimedica	CORACTO		Bioabsorbable	Rapamycin		Submitted for CE Mark

Alvimedica	Santez	Bioabsorbable stent	Bioabsorbable	Unknown		
amg	ITRIX		Bioabsorbable	Rapamycin		
amg	PicoElite		Durable	Paclitaxel	NA	CE Mark approval gained
Atrium Medical	CINATRA DES		No polymer	ISA247 (voclosporin)		
Avantec	Duraflex DES		Durable	Pimecolimus		
B. Braun	Coroflex Please		Durable	Paclitaxel	NA	CE Mark approval gained
Balton	Luc-Chopin2		Bioabsorbable	Paclitaxel	NA	CE Mark approval gained
Biosensors	Axxion		No polymer	Paclitaxel	NA	CE Mark approval gained
Biosensors	BioMatrix		Bioabsorbable	Biolimus A9	Clinical studies planned	CE Mark approval gained
Biosensors	BioMatrix Bifurcation	Bifurcation lesions	Not known	Biolimus A9		CE Mark approval gained

(Continued)

Company	Product Name	Notes	Polymer Type	Drug	Status US	Status OUS
Biosensors	Bioresorbable stent	Bioabsorbable stent	Not known	Unknown		
BIOTRONIK	Bioabsorbable metal stent		None	Pimecolimus		
BIOTRONIK	ProGenic		Durable	Pimecolimus		
Boston Scientific	Evolution	Abluminal coating	Bioabsorbable	Everolimus		
Boston Scientific	LabCoat	Abluminal coating	Bioabsorbable	Paclitaxel		
Boston Scientific	PROMUS		Durable	Everolimus	On the market	CE Mark approval gained
Boston Scientific	PROMUS Element		Durable	Everolimus	US clinical trial under way	OUS clinical trial under way
Boston Scientific	TAXUS Petal	Bifurcation lesions	Durable	Paclitaxel		
Boston Scientific	TAXUS Element		Durable	Paclitaxel	US clinical trial enrollment complete	OUS clinical trial enrollment complete

Boston Scientific	TAXUS Liberté		Durable	Paclitaxel	On the market	CE Mark approval gained
Boston Scientific	TAXUS Express		Durable	Paclitaxel	On the market	CE Mark approval gained
Boston Scientific	Bioabsorbable polymer stent	Bioabsorbable stent	Bioabsorbable	Paclitaxel / Everolimus		
Boston Scientific	Bioabsorbable metal stent	Bioabsorbable stent	Bioabsorbable	Paclitaxel / Everolimus		
CardioMind	Sparrow	Small vessels	Bioabsorbable	Sirolimus		
Cardiotec	Cilotax		Bioabsorbable	Cilostazol & paclitaxel		
CID	Janus		No polymer	Tacrolimus	NA	CE Mark approval gained
CID	Janus Flex		No polymer	Tacrolimus	NA	CE Mark approval gained
CID	OPTIMA		No polymer	Tacrolimus	NA	CE Mark approval gained
CID	Sculptured DES	Abluminal reservoirs	No polymer			

(Continued)

Company	Product Name	Notes	Polymer Type	Drug	Status US	Status OUS
ClearStream	Intrepide		Durable	Trapidil	NA	CE Mark approval gained
Clinical Data, Inc.	ATL-146e DES		Durable	ATL-146e, a coronary vasodilator, and a type IV PDE inhibitor		
Cordis	Cordis Bifurcation	Bifurcation lesions	Not known			
Cordis	NEVO	Abluminal reservoirs	Bioabsorbable	Sirolimus		
Cordis	CYPHER		Durable	Sirolimus	On the market	CE Mark approval gained
Cordis	CYPHER-Select Plus		Durable	Sirolimus	NA	CE Mark approval gained
Cordis	CYPHER Anti-Thrombotic	Abluminal reservoirs	Bioabsorbable	Sirolimus & an antithrombotic agent		

Cordynamic	Active		Durable	Paclitaxel	NA	CE Mark approval gained
Cordynamic	IRIST		Durable	Triflusal and simvastatin	NA	Submitted for CE Mark
CorNova	CorNova DES		Durable	Generic drug		
Debiotech SA	Debiostent	Ceramic polymer	Durable	Unknown		
Devax	AXXESS	Bifurcation lesions	Bioabsorbable	Biolimus A9	US IDE study protocol approved	Submitted for CE Mark
Devax	Axxess LM	Left main lesions	Bioabsorbable	Biolimus A9		
DISA	Stellium		Bioabsorbable	Paclitaxel	NA	FIM study completed
Elixir	Epitome (Bioabsorbable)		Bioabsorbable	Myolimus	NA	FIM study completed
Elixir	Epitome (Durable)		Durable	Myolimus	NA	FIM study completed

(Continued)

57

Company	Product Name	Notes	Polymer Type	Drug	Status US	Status OUS
Elixir	Elixir BDES	Bioabsorbable stent	Bioabsorbable	Myolimus		
Elixir	Excella-bioabsorbable polymer		Bioabsorbable	Novolimus	NA	Clinical trial planned
Elixir	Excella-durable polymer		Durable	Novolimus	NA	CE Mark trial complete
Estracure	Estracure DES		Bioabsorbable	17-beta-estradiol		International pilot completed
Eucatech	Euca TAX		Bioabsorbable	Paclitaxel	NA	CE Mark approval gained
EuroCOR	AG 1295		Bioabsorbable	Tyrphostin AG 1295		
EuroCOR	PRONO		Not known	17-beta-estradiol	NA	International clinical study under way
EuroCOR	TAXCOR		Bioabsorbable	Paclitaxel	NA	CE Mark approval gained

EuroCOR	TAXCOR Polymer-Free	No polymer	Paclitaxel	NA	CE Mark approval gained
Global Therapeutics	Silencer	No polymer	Antisense		International clinical trial enrollment completed
Globamed	Omega	No polymer	Paclitaxel	NA	On market internationally, not in Europe
IBS	MAR-Tyn	Not known	Titanium nitrate-coated cobalt–chromium stent		
ICON	Nuloy DES	Bioabsorbable	Deforolimus		
InSitu Technologies	Monarch	Durable	Paclitaxel	NA	International clinical study under way
InSitu Technologies	Solus	Durable	Echinomycin	NA	
Intek	Apollo	Durable	Paclitaxel	NA	CE Mark approval gained

(Continued)

Company	Product Name	Notes	Polymer Type	Drug	Status US	Status OUS
ITGI Medical	Over & Under DES		No polymer	Covered with heterologous bovine pericardium		
JW Medical	Excel		Bioabsorbable	Sirolimus	NA	On market internationally, not in Europe
Kaneka	MAHOROBA		Bioabsorbable	Tacrolimus	NA	
Lepu	PARTNER	Bifurcation lesions	Durable	Sirolimus	NA	On market internationally, not in Europe
Lumen Therapeutics	LT-1942 DES		Not known	Oligo-L-arginine		
Medinol	573 DES		No polymer	Deforolimus		
Medlogics	COBRA-CCVT Biopolymer		Bioabsorbable	Cerivastatin		
Medlogics	COBRA-P Synergy		No polymer	Paclitaxel		

Medtronic	Endeavor	Durable	Zotarolimus	On the market	CE Mark approval gained
Medtronic	Endeavor Resolute	Durable	Zotarolimus	US clinical trial under way	CE Mark approval gained
Medtronic	Medtronic BAS	Bioabsorbable	Zotarolimus		
MeoMedical	Meo:DrugStar ST	Durable	Paclitaxel	NA	
Micell	MiStent	Bioabsorbable	Crystalline sirolimus		
MicroPort	FireBird	Durable	Sirolimus	NA	On the market outside Europe and U.S.
MicroPort	FireBird 2	Durable	Sirolimus	NA	On the market internationally
MicroPort	Mytrolimus-eluting stent	Durable	Mytrolimus		
Millimed	Millimed DES	Not known	Nitric oxide		
Minvasys	Amazonia PAX	No polymer	Paclitaxel	NA	

(Continued)

Company	Product Name	Notes	Polymer Type	Drug	Status US	Status OUS
Minvasys	Nile Pax and Delta Pax	Bifurcation lesions	No polymer	Paclitaxel	NA	
MIVT	VESTAsync		No polymer	Sirolimus	Clinical studies planned	CE Mark trial under way
Orbus	Genous		No polymer	Bioengineered surface technology	NA	CE Mark approval gained
Relisys	Corel+C		No polymer	Paclitaxel		
Relisys	Release-T		Durable	Paclitaxel	NA	International clinical trial enrollment completed
Sahajanand	Genistein-Sirolimus DES		Bioabsorbable	Genistein and sirolimus		
Sahajanand	Infinnium		Bioabsorbable	Paclitaxel	NA	CE Mark approval gained
Sahajanand	Infinnium-Core		Bioabsorbable	Paclitaxel	NA	International study under way

Sahajanand	Supra-Core		Bioabsorbable	Sirolimus	NA		International study under way
Sahajanand	Supralimus		Bioabsorbable	Sirolimus	NA		CE Mark approval gained
Sahajanand	Synchronnium		Bioabsorbable	Heparin and sirolimus	NA		
Sahajanand	Synchronnium Plus		Bioabsorbable	Heparin and sirolimus			
Stentys	Bifurcation DES	Bifurcation lesions	Durable	Paclitaxel			
Svelte	Svelte DES		No polymer	Limus family	In development		
Terumo Interventional	NOBORI		Bioabsorbable	Biolimus A9	NA		CE Mark approval gained
Tianjian	ProStent		Not known	Rapamycin	NA		International clinical study under way

(Continued)

Company	Product Name	Notes	Polymer Type	Drug	Status US	Status OUS
Translumina	YUKON Choice		No polymer	Sirolimus, rapamycin, 17-beta-estradiol; physicians choose drug & coat stent themselves	NA	CE Mark approval gained
Vascular Concepts	PRO COMM		Durable	Cyclosporine and sirolimus	NA	CE Mark trial under way
Vascular Concepts	ProNOVA		Durable	Sirolimus	NA	Submitted for CE Mark
Vascular Concepts	ProTAXX		Bioabsorbable	Paclitaxel	NA	CE Mark approval gained
VasoTech	PowerStent		Bioabsorbable	Anti-restenosis drug formulation		
X-Cell	ETHOS III		Bioabsorbable	17-beta-estradiol	Clinical studies planned	International clinical studies under way
Xtent	Custom NX		Bioabsorbable	Biolimus A9	NA	May no longer be in development